WHAT TO DO AFTER HEARING, "YOU HAVE MS?!" (MULTIPLE SCLEROSIS)

What To Do After Hearing, "You Have MS?!" (Multiple Sclerosis)

40 Ideas to Normalize Life When Not in Remission

Stephen J. Lally

Illustrations by Chris Purcell and Dyshon Smith

Foreword by Richard Buckler, Neurologist

To order additional copies of this book, contact:
Xlibris LLC
1-888-795-4274
www.Xlibris.com
Orders@Xlibris.com
142714

CONTENTS

Acknowledgments

To Lorie Elizabeth-Reese, for believing in me.

To Christopher Andrew Francis for his honesty and courage.

To Timothy Joseph and Patty Jane for their love, patience, and perseverance.

To my mom and dad for being them.

To my doctors, Richard Buckler and Lawrence Miller, for talking to me when I needed to talk.

To Denise for being a really good friend.

FOREWORD

As Steve Lally states in his book, "I needed to do what I could do and move on with my life". This was some of the advice I provided Steve after he was diagnosed with Multiple Sclerosis. I believe Steve's positive attitude and active life style has allowed him to contend with this condition and lead a full life. He does not allow this disease to interfere with his role as a father, counselor and man of faith.

This book is a way for Steve to help others with MS deal with this condition. His 40 ideas are positive, helpful activities that should assist all individuals with MS. I believe this book will be a very helpful guide for individuals and their families to cope with this disease. The activities are healthy for both the mind and body.

It has been my pleasure and honor to assist Steve in dealing with this illness. His attitude and ideas should be an inspiration for all MS patients. My hope is that the medical profession will continue to make advances in the treatment of this illness so we can help Steve and all individuals conquer this disease. This book should be a positive influence for all individuals with MS.

Richard A. Buckler, MD

INTRODUCTION

If it's not in remission, I don't have to tell you how debilitating multiple sclerosis can be. The purpose of this book is to take away some of the power MS has over us, if only for the time it took me to write this and you to read it. The goal is to extend that time for as long as possible, helping to create a satisfactory quality of life for you and other people living with this disease. I don't pretend to have a monopoly on the things one can do to get and feel better; however, after fifteen—make that sixteen years of tribulations and trials, I'm offering help and in a manner that is both effective and fun. This book is for YOU.

CHAPTER 1

THE ONSET

I recently found out that my nephew Matt contracted MS. As you may have already guessed, I have it, as well as my oldest sister, Pat. The neurologist explained that it is not hereditary but that there is a high rate of incidence in families. Is there really a difference? While not understanding his explanation, I have so many questions, not to mention fears, and I'm wondering if you do too. I've decided to write this book for Matt, for you, and for the countless others living with this disease. May you find hope, encouragement, and the ability to stay well.

I was diagnosed in November of '97 after two weeks of testing that seemed like two years. The doctors appeared to be as confused as I was, and that frightened me. I was reeling since the initial diagnosis, optical neuritis, and felt horrible most of the time. Looking back, I had symptoms most of my life, but I never took the time to investigate what was really going on. After going temporarily blind on the golf course (boy, do I miss golf), seeing my doctor (who did a nice job of telling me nothing), being sent to an ophthalmologist (I think it's an eye doctor), being redirected to a specialist (and what I asked, he didn't answer), and finally going to a neurologist (I knew I was in trouble), I went through a battery of tests at each stop. The ruling-out period ended, and the survey said (remember that game show *Family Feud* with Richard Dawson as host?) MULTIPLE SCLEROSIS. I didn't clap. Nobody clapped. I didn't know what it was. I was glad they, the doctors, knew what it was, or I thought they knew what it was. I probably don't have to tell you how devastating it was to learn that they didn't know what it was and that there wasn't, and still isn't, a cure. I had no idea how to talk about what I was feeling. I also wasn't sure if anyone would understand.

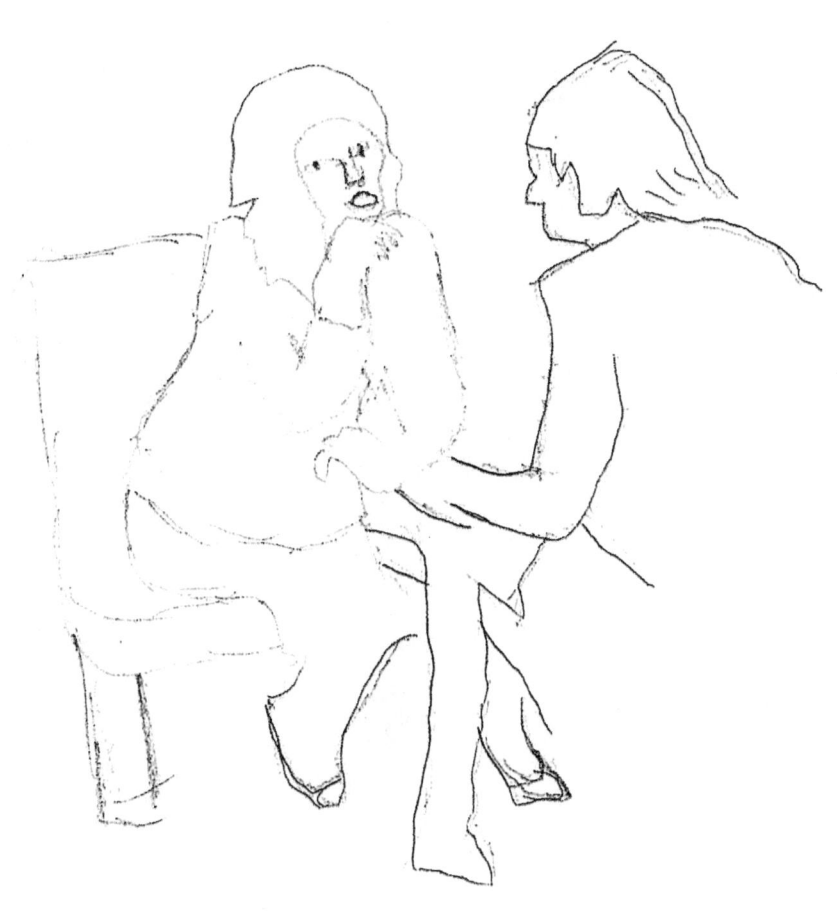

CHAPTER 2

BIOLOGICALLY SPEAKING

The neurologist explained that there were three medications on the market with FDA approval, all having about a 33 percent chance of working or being effective. I had a very difficult time in understanding that the medicine treats symptoms only. He went on to say that if I was lucky enough to be one of the 33 percent, it could reduce the rate of relapse by maybe 35 to 40 percent. I didn't like the numbers. I'm embarrassed to tell you that I turned down the medicine! For the rest of '97 and all of '98, I was in and out of the hospital a couple of times. In January of '99, I crawled back to his office, asking if I could try the medicine. He didn't turn me down. So I started taking medication, and after discovering through trial and error what actually worked, I began to get results and gain some degree of stability. Dr. Buckler, the neurologist, also helped me understand how the medication worked with the following example. He explained that MS is similar to a virus running around the body and feeding on myelin sheaths, which wrap our nerves. He continued to explain that the medication was made up of the same molecular structure as the myelin sheaths, acting as a decoy and hoping the MS attacks it and leaves the nerves alone. This example renewed my faith in the hope that one day, an actual cure will be found.

So the first item on the list of forty ideas to normalize life when not in remission is "TAKE YOUR MEDICINE"!

Soon after beginning medication, my mother-in-law at the time suggested that I go see a nutritionist. I was surprised to find out that he knew as much as if not more than the neurologist. Time has taught me that it's all about perspective from the model one utilizes. For example, a doctor comes from a medical model compared to a nutritionist using a nutritional or holistic approach toward treating a disease. The nutritionist explained that MS results from a deficiency in the immune system—that it attacks itself for unknown reasons, resulting in the body not being able to protect it from infection or disease. He further explained that if we feed the body what it needs, such an effort could result in good health. So he laid out a certain diet coupled with vitamins and supplements, suggesting that I give it some time for results to start taking place. The results have varied. I've had years of complete remission while the opposite has also been true.

"WATCH YOUR DIET" (including vitamins and supplements) is the second item on the list of forty ideas to normalize life when not in

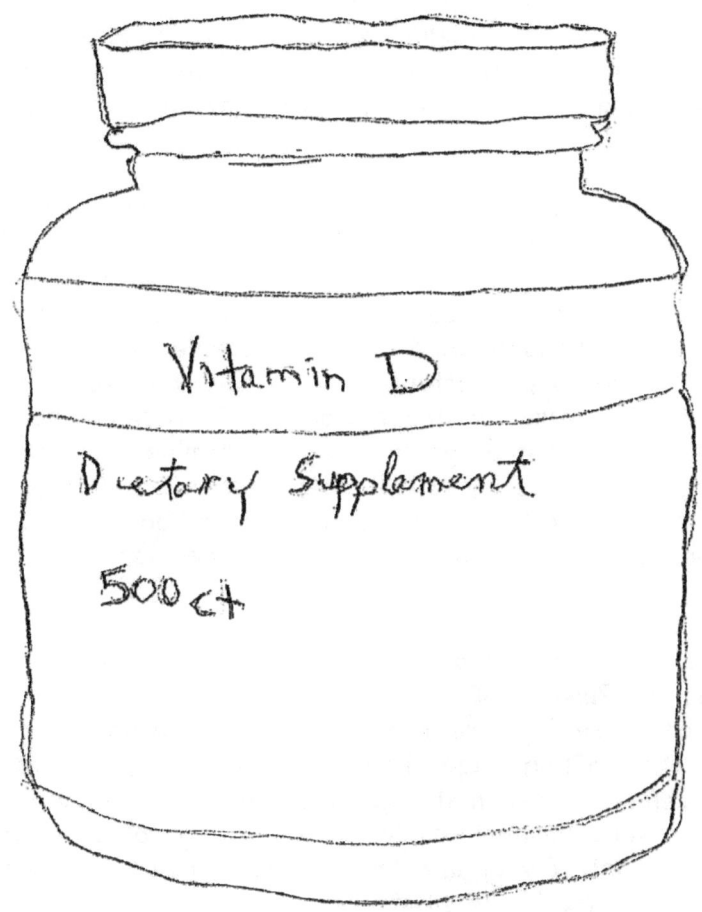

Keeping with the theme of "biologically speaking," the third item on the list of forty ideas to normalize life when not in remission is EXERCISE!

There is one rule that you must adhere to: Don't be a hero. You know how easy it is to get hurt without doing anything, so please be very careful. There might be times when symptoms get exacerbated after exercising, but don't let that fool you. Exercise is a good thing, so try not to talk yourself out of doing it. I'm guessing you know that feeling of breaking a good sweat after a nice jog or run. Also, be sure to stretch before engaging in this activity. Try and push yourself a little bit, but always remember rule number 1.

Number 4 on the list of forty ideas to normalize life when not in remission is "GO TO A BATTING CAGE"!

You have to really like baseball to engage in this one! It's a combination of exercise and fun. This activity is about hitting baseballs or softballs pitched from a machine, in case you didn't know. One thing to pay attention to is how long you stay in the cage. Where I'm from, for about a dollar, you receive about fifteen balls. The level of your progression will determine how long you can stay in the cage. Years ago, I was able to stay in the cage for more than one round, but today, not so much. Your body will tell you so. If you engage, take care of yourself, and remember, wear a helmet!

Number 5 on the list of forty ideas to normalize life when not in remission is "PLAY BASEBALL"!

It made sense to place this item here, thinking about it after going to the batting cage. This idea might require people who have the same interest in the game. If you want to keep it simple, playing backyard baseball could be the thing to do, especially if children are part of your life. Simply playing catch with someone is another option. You decide what works for you!

Number 6 on the list of forty ideas to normalize life when not in remission is "PLAY BASKETBALL"!

In case you haven't noticed, I tend to correlate exercise with playing sports. Sometime after being diagnosed, I remembered that my legs would go dead while playing basketball. It didn't happen often, but knowing what I know now, it was probably one of my first symptoms. Anyway, I want to tell you about this game called Around the World. The idea is to make it to the other side of the lane opposite of where you start (see picture). Start at one side of the lane on or close to the first block or dash. You get two chances at every shot. If you make it the first time, move on to the next block or dash. If you miss, you get to "chance" it—meaning you get to shoot again. If you miss the chance, you go back to the beginning and you start all over. Make sure you stop at the foul line and shoot from there before going to the opposite side. The first person who gets around the entire lane puts themselves in a position to win; however, you have to make a three-point shot (see picture again) to win. Remember, everybody wins! It can be a lot of fun! One of my goals is to organize a fund-raiser called Around the World for MS by utilizing this game. I'll keep you posted.

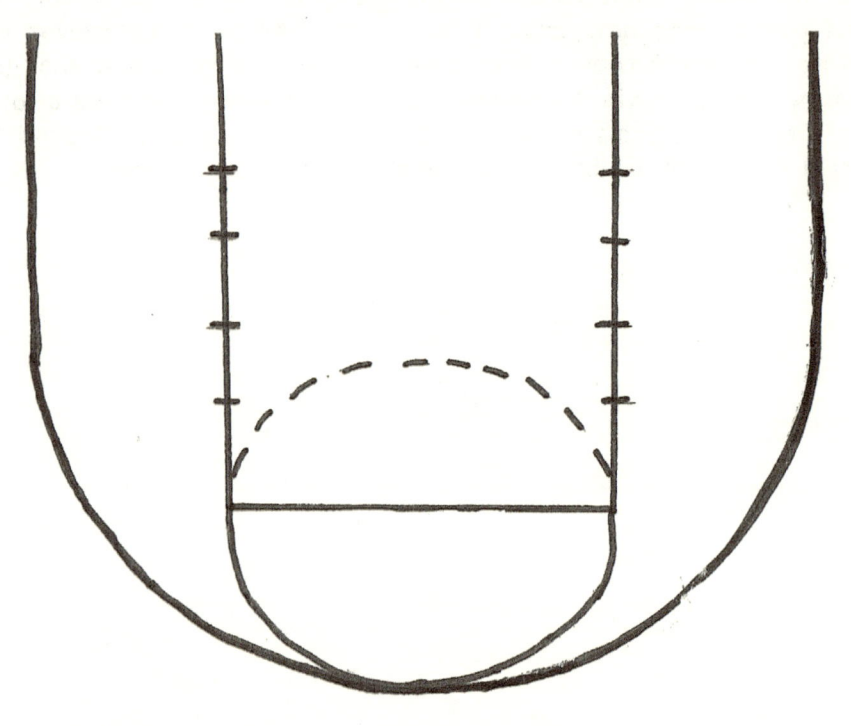

Number 7 on the list of forty ideas to normalize life when not in remission is "THROW A FOOTBALL"!

I guess you can throw a football without someone else, but then you have no one to throw it back! I suggest you find someone who has a similar interest. I'd like to tell you about a game that my son Chris came up with. Go to a field—it doesn't even have to be a football field—and determine the goal lines. Go from one end of the field to the other, throwing and catching. Since I can't run anymore, Chris was doing most of the running. It's one of those games where you get to be the player you want to be on the team you want to be. It's pretty awesome. It does end up being a nice workout for Chris, and I get to see where I'm at physically. Hope you got a visual!

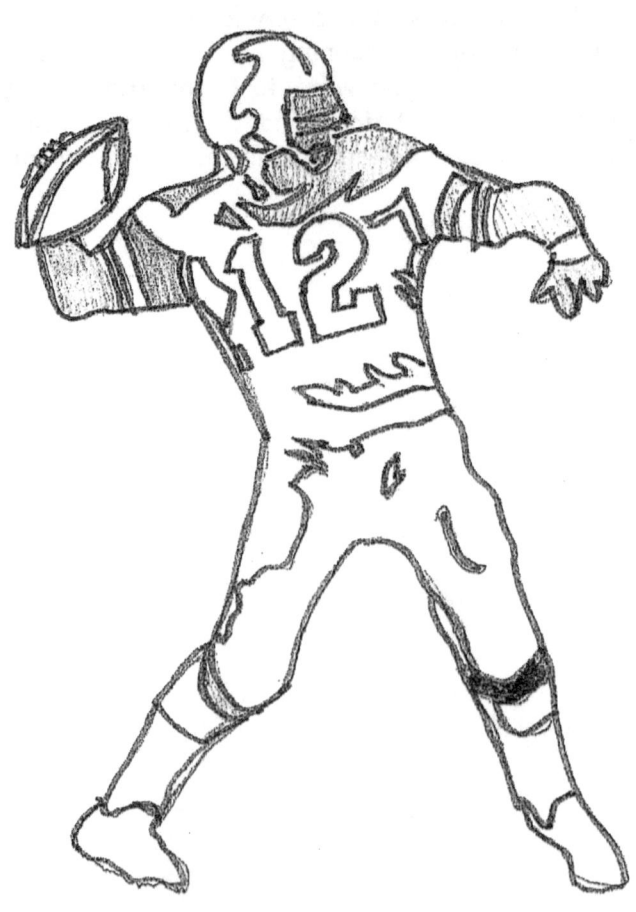

I'm not so sure if this next item is a sport; however, number 8 on the list of forty ideas is "PLAY PUTT-PUTT."

This activity can be a lot of fun; however, it can also take a lot out of you physically. If you have kids, it's certainly something to at least think about doing. It can also be pretty wonderful playing with a significant other. One thing that I do recommend is to NOT keep score. One school of thought is that the person with the most hole in ones wins! And honestly, after it's over, we all get ice cream. So don't spend too much money, but go have some fun when you can. And remember to sit down when you have to.

Number 9 on the list of forty ideas is "WALK A DOG"!

I'm pretty sure this is not a sport, but it sure feels like it. Even when I wasn't feeling too well, I made it a point to take my dog, Sparky, out for a walk. He always made me smile, and I know we got closer. Divorce has taken a lot of things away from me, and Sparky is one of them. I miss him so much. Is there such a thing as pet-walking services? I hope so. If it can't be Sparky, maybe it could be another pug. Did I tell you that Sparky is a pug?

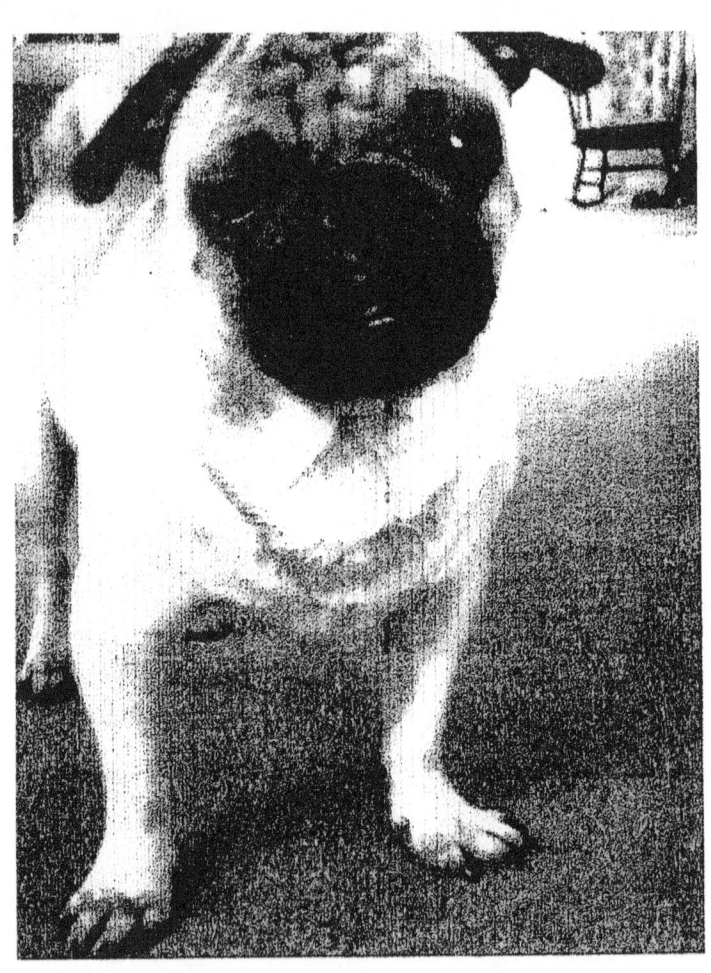

Number 10 on the list of forty ideas is "PLAY PING-PONG"!

One Christmas, I went out and bought a table, and it stayed in the dining room for close to a year. Did you know it is an Olympic sport? This activity can be a little deceiving. It takes more out of you than you might think. Be careful not to extend yourself too much. It also might be a good idea to shorten the game by reducing the score. Usually, a game goes to 21. Maybe you end it earlier when not feeling well. Volley for serve!?

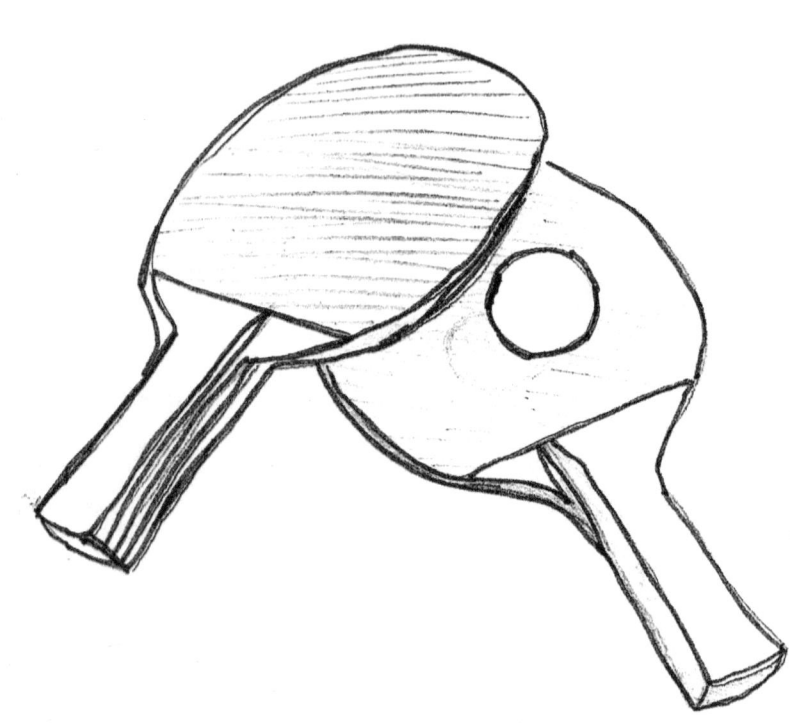

Number 11 on the list is "PLAY GOLF"!

I can't believe I put this on the list. It's something I would really struggle to do right now physically. I can hit some balls from a practice range, but even that doesn't last too long. I don't have enough strength or stamina to play anymore, and I'm really upset about it. So what does one do? When my kids tell me that they want to hit golf balls, boy, do I start looking for my clubs! After finding them and some for the kids, off to the golf range we go! I discovered that being together and hitting balls with them is as good as if not better than playing a round of golf. Another valuable lesson learned. My neurologist told me years ago that I needed to do what I could do and move on with my life. Thank you, Dr. Buckler.

CHAPTER 3

PSYCHOLOGICALLY SPEAKING

This chapter is tailor-made for you, offering opportunities to take care of yourself and, hopefully, discover something new about yourself. Let me know what you find.

Number 12 on the list is "READ A BOOK"!

It doesn't have to be a book with a story to it; it can be a book based on fact or fiction if it does. It can be anything that interests you—affirmations, poetry, or how about an autobiography? One on my favorites is *Chicken Soup for the Recovering Soul*. It's filled with personal stories of healing. After reading it, I found myself thinking that some of those people would trade places with me in a minute. I don't mean to minimize our situation, but we are not alone regarding pain and hardship. Try and find a book that will take YOU out of you.

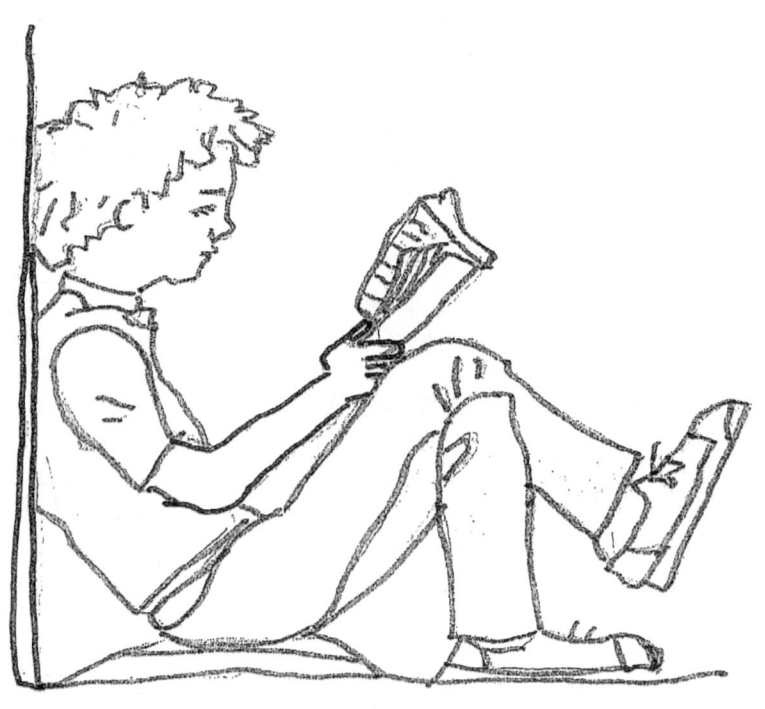

Number 13 on the list is "TELL SOMEBODY HOW YOU FEEL"!

This can be a difficult thing, depending on the kind of person you are. Culture might have something to do with it as well. I grew up in a family and neighborhood where one didn't ask for help. After the diagnosis, I found myself isolating from other people, feeling ashamed, like I did something wrong. How crazy is that? You need to know that you didn't do anything wrong. You also need to know that it can be a disease of isolation if you allow it to be. Today, tell somebody how you feel; it's one way to get better.

Number 14 is "MAKE YOUR OWN T-SHIRT"!

This idea is a combination of fun and building up self-esteem. I have about five or six new Ts due to this activity. Making a T-shirt can be about anything you want it to be. Mine was about sports—surprise, surprise. It doesn't have to be expensive either. You don't need to purchase new T-shirts; just use existing ones! You will probably have to go out and buy the letters and numbers, but even that can be fun. I ended up looking for such items in an arts-and-crafts store, and it turned into so much more. The conversations that take place after people see the T-shirt you create will be worth the effort. Let me know.

Number 15 is "KEEP A JOURNAL"!

This used to read as "Keep a journal of your feelings." After talking with others, it was decided that the idea of keeping a journal about feelings could be counterproductive. As we all know, it's tough enough to live with MS on a daily basis, let alone revisiting it by writing down how one feels (although I believe it has its place). So now, just write what you want, whether it's a feeling, an idea, or maybe a to-do list—whatever you think will work for you. Don't forget a pen or pencil.

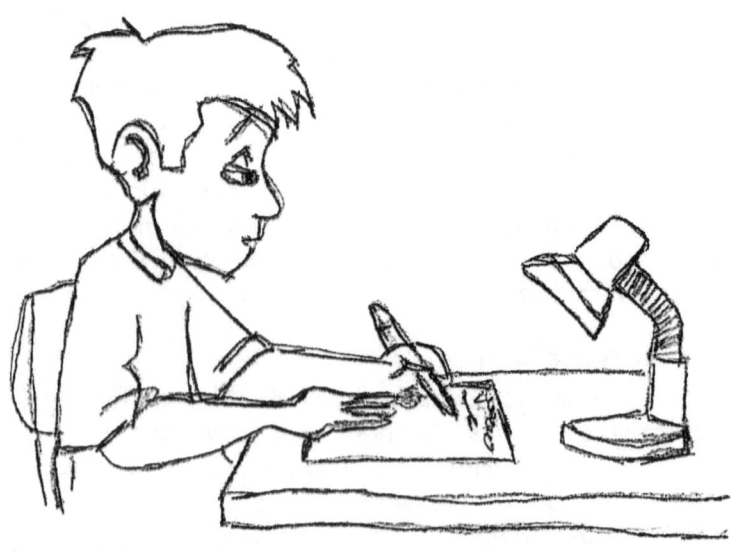

Number 16 is "DO YOUR LAUNDRY"!

It might not be the most popular item on the list, but you'll be clean, and you'll feel good about yourself! This idea is not so much about doing the laundry as it is about being able to and having fun doing it! One way to do this is listening to your favorite radio station or maybe a CD of your favorite band. Wow, I'm really behind the times. Today, I guess it's more about downloading your favorite music on an iPod or some other electronic device. You could also talk to somebody on a cell or telephone via speaker, accomplishing two things at one time. Sometimes, I have to go to a Laundromat, and it almost forces me to talk to people, whether I want to or not. I guess things could be worse. Don't forget the fabric softener!

This next idea could be at the root of "psychologically speaking." Number 17 on the list is "ASK FOR HELP"!

I think that when we are able to ask for help, it speaks volumes about our self-worth. I probably don't have to remind you that I'm the guy who first turned down the medicine! For some reason, I like to carry laundry down three flights of stairs just to prove to myself that I can. My roommate at the time brought it to my attention that I was putting myself in a position to get hurt. Another person explained that I was taking something away from other people by not asking them for help. I learned that asking for help is reciprocal—as in both parties benefiting. Think of a situation where you could ask for help. Don't let your pride get in the way.

Now to get silly. Number 18 on the list is "SING A SONG"!

Did you ever watch a sporting event or some type of performance where they played and/or sang a rendition of the "Star-Spangled Banner"? Tell me you never said to yourself or out loud, "I can do better than that"? I decided to see if I could do exactly that! With a former girlfriend's help, I sang at a Little League baseball all-star game and at a Pop Warner game as her children participated in both sports. Now, you don't have to do this activity in a public forum; that's just how it happened for me. Maybe for you, it's in the shower or in the car. Wherever it is, take a risk, have some fun, and sing a song.

To stay silly, number 19 on the list is "WRITE A SONG"!

Have you ever written a song or tried to write a song? I recently wrote my first song, and I believe my inspiration came from a . . . I wanted to do something as a way to say thank you, and I began to write. I didn't know where it was going as it turned into a song! I call it "Days of Grace."

started with a dream,
turned into desire,
quickly changed to action,
my heart caught on fire.

(refrain) on the first day of grace,
new things take their place;
incredible it seems.
it started with a dream.

so my heart caught on fire,
heard You call my name;
prayer and meditation,
things haven't been the same.

(refrain) on the second day of grace,
I think I pulled the ace;
incredible it seems.
it started with a dream.

things haven't been the same,
then She came along;
believe me when I tell you,
She's the fairest of them all.

(refrain) on the third day of grace,
I tried to get to first base;
incredible it seems.
it started with a dream.

the fairest of them all,
We held each other's hand;
shared our past and pain.
will it be forged in sand?

(refrain) on the fourth day of grace,
I think We have a case;
incredible it seems.
it started with a dream.

That's it for the verses; the rest are all refrains, and I decided to throw in some fun.

on the fifth day of grace,
tell it to my face;
incredible it seems.
it started with a dream.

on the sixth day of grace,
what are you doing with that can of Mace?
incredible it seems.
it started with a dream.

on the seventh day of grace,
we think the wabbit won the wace;
incredible it seems.
it started with a dream.

on the eighth day of grace,
I really love this place;
incredible it seems.
it started with a dream.

The song ends with the first verse.

started with a dream,
turned into desire,
quickly changed to action,
my heart caught on fire.

What do you think? Please let me know. I'm also interested to hear if you have any questions about the song.

Number 20 on the list of forty ideas is "MAKE A COLLAGE"!

This is one idea where you may discover something about yourself. For this activity, you will need to get some magazines, a pair of scissors, and paper or poster board. You'll also need tape or glue. You can do this in a couple of different ways. One is individually; another is in a group. I remember that when my mother-in-law passed away, I made a collage in honor of her memory. I ended up getting it framed and hanging it on the living-room wall for the longest time. If you ever engaged in group therapy, it would surprise me to hear that you never participated in such an activity. There are different ways to discuss the work being done; one is to ask each other what one sees. It might produce something interesting, and it certainly should be fun. Let me know if I can help in any way.

CHAPTER 4

SOCIALLY SPEAKING

This is a chapter where connecting with other people and maintaining the relationship is the ideal.

Number 21 on the list of forty ideas is "WATCH YOUR FAVORITE TV SHOW"!

I believe this belongs in this category, but I'm not convinced it doesn't belong somewhere else. Let me know what you think. The thought is that you will be watching TV with someone else, not alone. Honestly, I don't have a favorite TV show. My oldest son, Chris, has one, *The Big Bang Theory*, and he has invited me to sit down and watch it on occasion. Besides it being a great show, it's great to see and hear him laugh so much. As a divorced father without primary custody, it feels like I miss out on so much.

Number 22 on the list of forty ideas is "WATCH A MOVIE"!

You can do this inside your own home, at a movie theater, or I guess, wherever. The suggestion is to engage in this activity with other people, although watching a movie by yourself can be really interesting. How about watching a movie with one of your favorite stars, like a Denzel Washington or a Hilary Swank? The type of movie you wish to watch could depend on your mood at the time, so try and figure out if it's action, drama, or adventure. You can throw romance into that as well. I'd like to put a plug-in for *A Little Bit of Heaven*. Check it out and let me know.

COLUMBIA

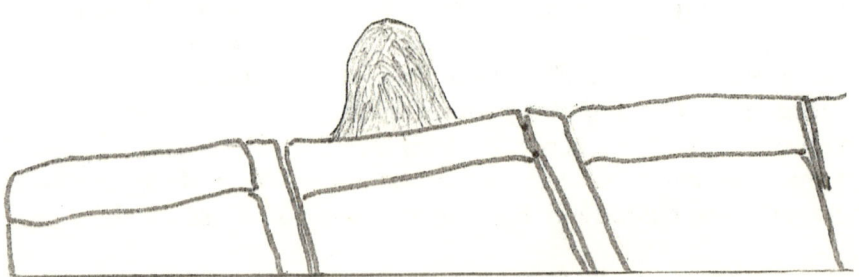

Number 23 on the list of forty ideas is "ASK SOMEBODY HOW THEY ARE FEELING"!

I was out shopping at a supermarket when I saw an old friend from college. She has MS, and she didn't look as well as she did the last time I saw her. The entire right side of her body was drooped over, and I knew something drastically changed. So I asked her what happened. I felt really dumb as she explained to me, "Nothing happened. It's the MS." I sometimes forget that it's the nature of the disease, how it can strike at any time. I was amazed at her strength as she described this experience. It helped me check myself and put things in a different perspective. People have as much difficulty as me, if not more. Today, remember to ask someone how they are feeling. Thank you, Michelle.

Number 24 on the list of forty ideas to normalize life when not in remission is "ATTEND A COMEDY CLUB."

You can do this in a couple of different ways. You can attend a show to watch others perform, or maybe you can be the performer. It shouldn't be too difficult to find a club in the area where you live. A warning I would like to give you is that not all establishments see a certain language as offensive. I think people disagree on what is considered offensive, so you will have to decide for yourself. If I could provide another suggestion, it would be to check out the club and see if you can tolerate the language and behavior. When I get up there (did I tell you I am going to get up there?), I'm going to keep it as clean as I can. I'll be in touch.

Number 25 on the list of forty ideas to normalize life when not in remission is "TEXT A FRIEND"!

I'm not a big fan of doing things electronically; however, I've learned that it has its place. I THINK I was one of the last people on earth to get a cell phone. I KNOW I was the last person to get a home computer. I probably shouldn't be proud of the fact that I made it through graduate school with ONLY a typewriter (I did use the school's computer on occasion). Anyway, when you're not feeling well enough to call and talk to someone, it's probably a good time to text. You can also text people on special occasions, like a birthday.

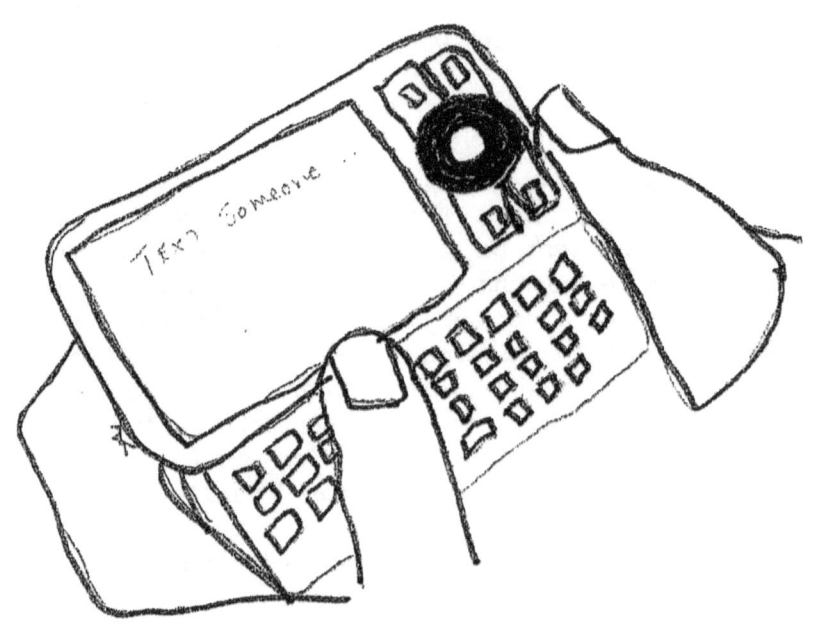

Number 26 on the list of forty ideas to normalize life when not in remission is "WRITE A LETTER"!

You don't necessarily need a reason to do this. Think of the people you haven't seen in a while and might not have the phone numbers of. Also think of the people that you have some unresolved conflicts with and don't know how to go about them. The timing of writing and sending a letter is important, but when in doubt, write! And did you ever write a letter to yourself? The reasons are many. Let me know if you need help.

Number 27 on the list of forty ideas to normalize life when not in remission is "PLAY A BOARD GAME"!

If I had to emphasize anything about this activity, it would be to just play and not worry so much about winning. This activity does include the element of spending time with family and friends, not that you can't include them in the other ideas. Another good thing is that you get to see a certain side of people you might not see—for example, what they laugh about, how they laugh, etc. The hardest part about this activity might be agreeing on which game to play! If that's the case, you know you're doing pretty well. I'd like to put a plug out there for Scrabble. How about you? What would be your choice of game? Let everybody know that the only rule is to be a good sport!

Number 28 on the list of forty ideas to normalize life when not in remission is "MAKE A BIRTHDAY CARD"!

Try not to think of this as a way out of buying a card. Try to think of the meaning it will have after you give it to someone. Depending on how artistic you are, you can do a lot with this activity. And how many times did you go to a store and find the perfect card that expressed all the things you ever wanted to say? How great would it be to be able to construct the same kind of card? So check your calendar, discover whose birthday is upcoming, and surprise someone. HAPPY BIRTHDAY!

Number 29 on the list of forty ideas to normalize life when not in remission is "CALL A FRIEND"!

Who do you need to call right now? Who needs to hear from you right now? I'm sure you know. Who would you like to hear from right now? This should make it a little easier as far as figuring out who to call. You don't necessarily have to have a reason. What would we do without friends? Make the call!

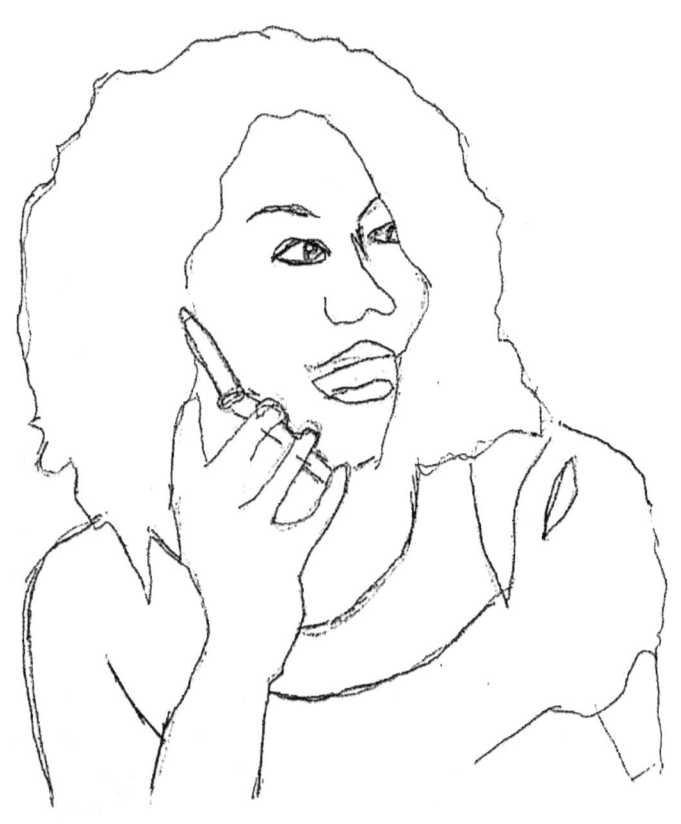

Number 30 on the list of forty ideas to normalize life when not in remission is "ATTEND AN OPEN MIKE NIGHT"!

Mike stands for microphone, in case you didn't know. Many restaurants and bars already offer this or are adding it to their weekly schedules. Most offer music, some provide comedy, and others give you the option. If you're not the type to jump up on stage and perform, maybe you could go to watch and enjoy. There's nothing like watching a friend perform and your being there to catch it. I think of getting up there one day, either to sing or do a short comedy routine. Wish me luck.

Number 31 on the list of forty ideas to normalize life when not in remission is "SEND AN E-MAIL."

My only rule about this is this: don't send information to family members that needs to be conveyed in person. I know this activity has its place, evident by people at work transferring necessary information. When did we confuse things by e-mailing feelings? I'm sure that is not what the founding fathers had in mind. E-mail when it's appropriate.

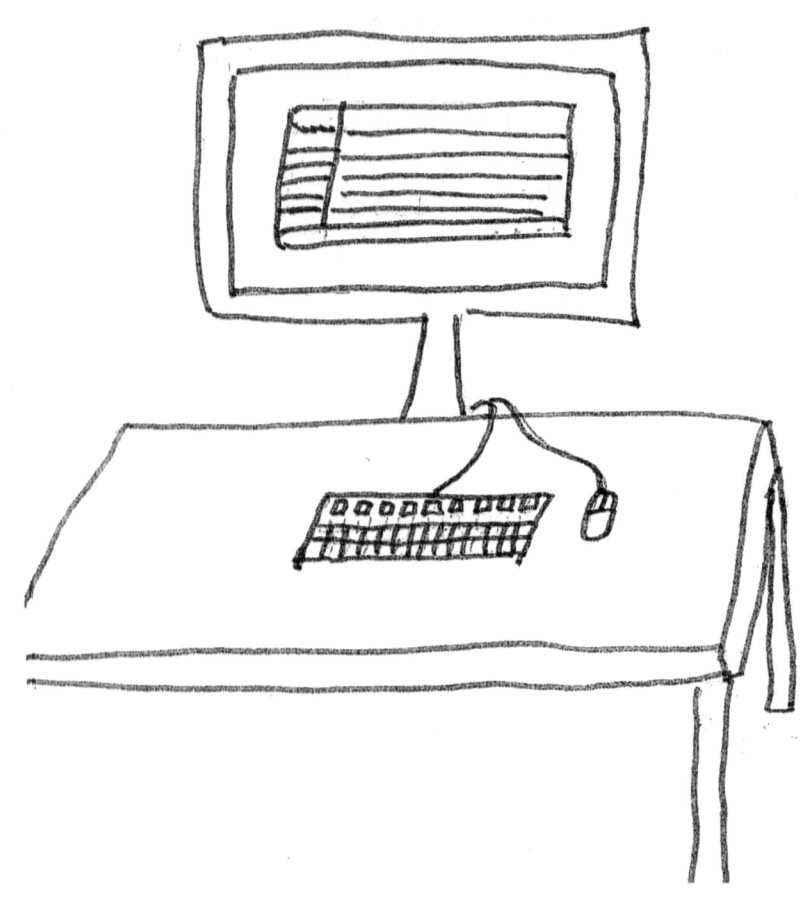

Number 32 on the list of forty ideas to normalize life when not in remission is "DO KARAOKE"!

You can do this a couple of different ways. One is to throw caution to the wind and just do it yourself, or you can sit back and watch other people. The trick is to be prepared if you decide to get up there and sing. Here's a helpful hint. Pick out a place where karaoke is an option and go there with no intention to participate; simply go and check things out. Determine if you would be comfortable and ask a lot of questions. You can't control everything, but I would try to have a say in some things you might get nervous about. You decide what your comfort level is, and the best part is, you get to pick out the song! Let me know how it goes.

Number 33 on the list of forty ideas is "TAKE A TRAIN RIDE"!

Honestly, I've taken only one train ride since my diagnosis, but boy, was it wonderful! I was with my two sons, my daughter, and one of their friends. They just loved looking out the window. We started about fifteen miles outside of Philadelphia and took the train to almost the center of the city. It was actually the last stop, so we got out, had some lunch, walked around, then came back home. The kids still talk about that trip. With the weather getting warmer, something tells me it might be time for another train ride.

Number 34 on the list of forty ideas is "VISIT A FRIEND"!

You decide how to do this activity based on how you're feeling. Unless somebody lived really close, I'd have to drive. I can last about a quarter of a mile if I have to walk anywhere. Riding a bicycle is another possibility; however, I learned the hard way that I have to bike back! Anyway, one thing I know is that the more I interact with people, the better I feel.

Number 35 on the list of forty ideas is "HAVE LUNCH WITH A FRIEND"!

There are some factors involved like money, time, and availability. Let's assume there are no obstacles getting in the way. Think of someone that you would like to have lunch with (it could also be breakfast or dinner) and attempt to contact them now or before the day ends! Most people won't follow through on such a thing; that's why I'm asking (telling) you to act now. And I know there's somebody out there that you need to catch up with! A lot could happen. Make a date.

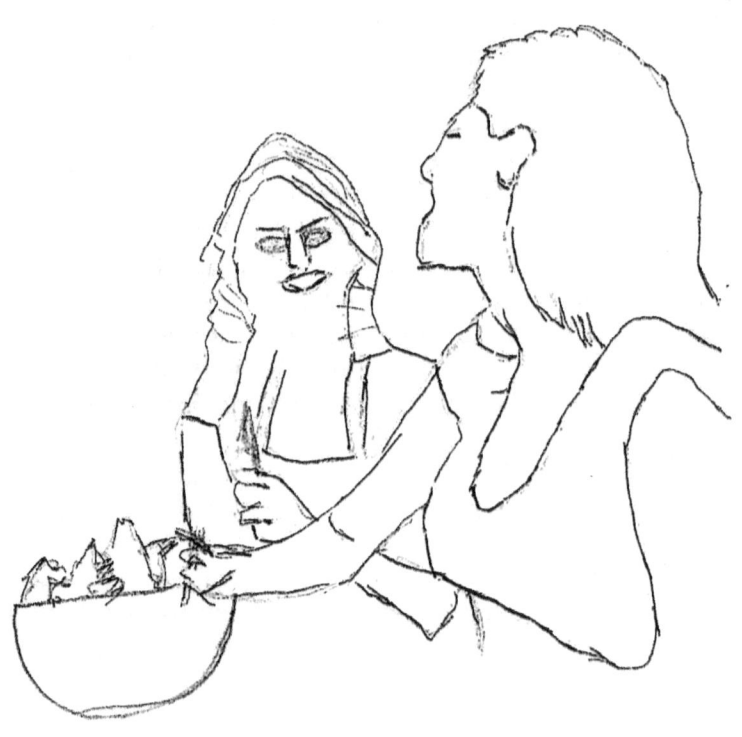

Number 36 on the list is "SHOP ONLINE"!

Honestly, I don't really know where this item belongs as far as the category, but this is where it placed!? I think that the last time I bought something for myself, it consisted of an ink cartridge for a printer. When I do shop online, it's usually for my children. In this world of electronics, one can do a lot on a computer, and shopping might as well be one of them, especially for people with MS. I'm sure you know the feeling of seeing somebody receive an item in the mail, whether they knew or not that it was coming. Nice job.

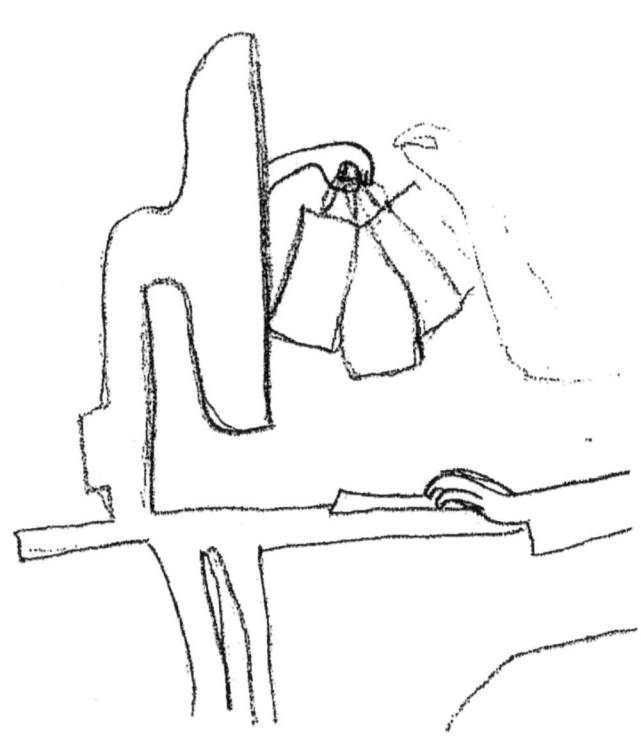

Number 37 on the list is "WORK THE SNACK STAND"!

This is all about connecting with people besides helping out somebody or something. If you don't have someone close to you playing some type of Little League baseball or football, you can always volunteer. From personal experience, it's such a pleasure serving children food or drink from a snack stand. The younger the cuter, if you know what I mean. I trust that you understand that you are going to be on your feet for a while, so be prepared! And you might as well check out the game before or after you put in your time. This activity forces you to talk and interact with people. It seems to have a way of presenting itself at the right time. Let me know if it happens like that.

Number 38 on the list is "ATTEND A COMMUNITY EVENT"!

There's a wide range of things to pick from. You could go to the movies, you could watch a play, or you could attend a concert or perhaps a sporting event. Personally, I like twelve-step meetings or a group that provides information sharing. Did you know that there are MS support groups? I'd be surprised if there wasn't one in your area. They're very helpful. I learned as much as if not more about living with MS from my group than I did from my doctors. I'd be interested to hear about what types of community events interest you. Talk to you soon.

Number 39 is "LEARN HOW TO DRAW"!

I was ready to accept the fact that I couldn't draw and figured it would stay that way. Then one day, I found myself sitting in an art class at an alternative school where I used to work. The teacher explained different ways of how to draw, and one of them was to simply look at a picture and draw it! To my surprise, the picture I drew came out okay, and it still hangs on my bedroom wall. Thank you, Nancy! Give yourself permission to draw even if you think you can't.

CHAPTER 5

SPIRITUALLY SPEAKING

Last but not least, number 40 is "FIND YOUR GOD"!

I want to make it clear that it is not my intention to push my beliefs on you—only to share my experience. Here goes. One day, a friend of mine, Chuck, asked me to sponsor him after deciding to convert to Catholicism. He explained that I needed to participate in the same requirements expected of him during his conversion. One night during an education class, the priest was discussing the seven sacraments of the Catholic faith—specifically, the Anointing of the Sick. My understanding of this was that it was designated for people about to die, possibly receiving the last rites or making a last confession. The priest helped me understand that the sacrament was available to anyone—Catholic, of course—suffering in any way and was looking for healing. We spoke after class about me having MS, and we set up an appointment for the very next day to receive the sacrament. I want to tell you that the Catholic faith is a sacramental faith where, upon receiving any of the seven sacraments, JESUS BECOMES PRESENT—LITERALLY PRESENT! I didn't really understand what this meant until I entered Father Joe's office the next day, and I could feel the energy. After the initial greeting, we got started. I remember praying together and listening to him read from the Bible. He anointed me with oil, specifically touching my hands and my head, then administered a blessing. The next thing I knew, Jesus was standing next to me. I'm going to say that again. JESUS WAS STANDING NEXT TO ME!

I was stunned. He asked if I would help Him carry the cross and said He would nail the MS to it after reaching Calvary. It was such an honor. I watched Him nail the MS to the cross after we arrived. We both stood there, watching it blow in the wind, like it was a flag or something. He then told me to "go in peace," and the next thing I knew, Father Joe was pushing on my shoulder, asking if everything was all right. It was more than all right. I was healed! I was MS-free for the next six or seven years until IT came back for reasons I now understand. I can't wait to share that story with you. Till then.

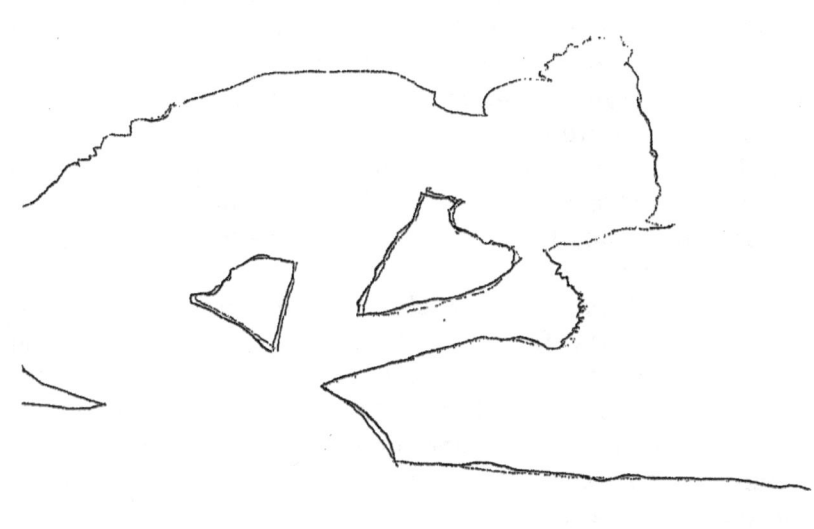

Anointing of the Sick

Part 2

Here is my understanding of why IT came back after six or seven years of remission. After moving into a new neighborhood, I set out to find the local Catholic church. Much to my surprise, I discovered that it was only a few blocks away from where I was about to live. I stopped by the rectory to find out the daily and Sunday Mass schedules and ended up talking with the pastor. I felt comfortable enough to ask him about the possibility of receiving the sacrament of the Anointing of the Sick, if possible. My thinking was that it was a one-and-done type of thing. Much to my surprise, the pastor told me that people receive it as often as needed. It surprised me even more when he asked if I wanted to receive it immediately. If you guessed that I turned him down, you would be correct! I seem to have developed a pattern of turning down things that are usually good for me. I did, however, end up scheduling an appointment for the following day.

So I headed over to the church the next day, and we went to a room separate from the sanctuary. After some small talk, the priest suggested that I get comfortable, and not too long afterward, he read from the Bible. Soon after that, he anointed me with oil on my hands and head. Last, he said some prayers and had me say some prayers, and it ended, or so I thought. He encouraged me to go sit in the church and reflect on what just happened. While sitting in the church, reflecting, the Mass started. I thought that it would interfere with my reflection, but the opposite became true. I continued reflecting while following the Mass, and it came time for Holy Communion, another sacrament that occurs during Mass where participants "receive Jesus." I chose not to receive that day but wanted to observe the ceremony, continuing to reflect. Next thing I knew, I heard His voice, and I knew He was present. He actually started a conversation with me, saying, "You believe I can heal you again, right?" I responded, "Sure, I do." He went on to ask me, "Would it be okay if I give the blessing to someone else who hasn't had it yet?" After a slight hesitation, I replied, "Sure, it . . . would." I remember feeling guilty about the hesitation. He then told me the name of the person (Daniel) who was going to be healed! He thanked me and was gone! He thanked me. It was the greatest feeling ever. It was one of those moments where I knew everything was going to be okay.

CONCLUSION

This concludes *What to Do after Hearing "You have MS!?"* Thank you so much for your time and consideration. It was an honor to share my life with you. I can only hope you get something out of this book. Most activities will require some effort on your part, so be careful on what you engage in. Please stay in touch, as will I. Till we meet again!

e-mail address:

steve_lally@yahoo.com

www.ingramcontent.com/pod-product-compliance
Lightning Source LLC
Chambersburg PA
CBHW021040180526
45163CB00005B/2214